THE LIVER HEALTH HANDBOOK

A Patient's Guide to Understanding and Reversing Liver Diseases

MILLER JAMES

TABLE OF CONTENTS

TABLE OF CONTENTS 1
    INTRODUCTION 4
        Why Your Liver Is Important 4
        How Liver Diseases Start 5
        How to Protect and Heal Your Liver 8
    PART 1: UNDERSTANDING THE LIVER 12
        CHAPTER 1: THE LIVER'S ROLE IN THE BODY 13
        Key Jobs of a Healthy Liver 13
        How the Liver Affects Your Overall Health 16
        CHAPTER 2: RECOGNIZING LIVER DISEASE.........20
        Early Warning Signs and Symptoms 20
        What Your Symptoms Might Mean 24
        CHAPTER 3: DIAGNOSING LIVER PROBLEMS.......28
        Bloodwork and Imaging Tests 28
        Understanding Biopsies and Other Tests 33
    PART 2: COMMON LIVER CONDITIONS 38
        CHAPTER 4: NON-ALCOHOLIC FATTY LIVER
        DISEASE (NAFLD) 39
        What Is NAFLD? 39
        Risk Factors and Symptoms 40

Lifestyle Strategies for Reversal 44

CHAPTER 5: ALCOHOL-RELATED LIVER DISEASE (ARLD) 50

How Alcohol Affects Your Liver 50

How to Treat and Recover from ARLD 54

CHAPTER 6: HEPATITIS 60

What is Hepatitis? 60

Causes, Symptoms, and Treatments 63

How to Prevent Hepatitis 66

CHAPTER 7: CIRRHOSIS 70

What is Cirrhosis? 70

What Causes Cirrhosis and What Can It Do? 71

How to Manage Cirrhosis 74

CHAPTER 8: LIVER CANCER 78

Types of Liver Cancer and What Makes Them Different 79

Early Signs and How to Detect Liver Cancer 81

Treatment Options for Liver Cancer 85

PART 3: LIVER-FRIENDLY DIET AND NUTRITION ... 89

CHAPTER 9: THE ROLE OF DIET IN LIVER HEALTH 90

How Nutrition Affects the Liver 91

Foods to Support Liver Function 93

Foods to Limit for Liver Health 96

CHAPTER 10: FOODS TO AVOID FOR A HEALTHY LIVER 99

Foods and Habits That Harm the Liver 100

Moderation Tips for Risky Foods 105
CHAPTER 11: MEAL PLANS AND RECIPES 108
　Liver-Friendly Meal Ideas 108
　Recipes to Help Your Liver Recover 112
CONCLUSION 117
　Practical Steps to Protect Your Liver 118
　Innovations in Liver Disease Management 122
　Final Thoughts 127

INTRODUCTION

The Liver Health Handbook: A Patient's Guide to Understanding and Reversing Liver Diseases

Why Your Liver Is Important

Your liver is one of the most amazing organs in your body. It does so many important jobs, like cleaning your blood, turning food into energy, storing vitamins, and helping you digest fat by making bile. Even though the liver can heal itself, it's not indestructible. Unhealthy habits, infections, and certain inherited conditions can hurt your liver.

The tricky thing about liver problems is that they often start quietly, without obvious symptoms. That's why taking care of your liver is so important. A healthy liver keeps the rest of your body working well—it helps balance your hormones, fight off illnesses, and so much more.

How Liver Diseases Start

Liver problems usually happen when something damages the liver over time. Here are some common causes:

Too much fat in the liver: This can happen if someone is overweight or has other health issues, like diabetes. It's called non-alcoholic fatty liver disease (NAFLD).

Drinking too much alcohol: This can lead to liver damage, like alcoholic hepatitis or cirrhosis.

Viral infections: Diseases like hepatitis A, B, and C can harm liver cells.

Autoimmune problems: Sometimes, the body's immune system attacks the liver by mistake.

Inherited conditions: Diseases like hemochromatosis (too much iron) or Wilson's disease (too much copper) can damage the liver.

If these problems aren't treated, they can cause scarring, called fibrosis. Over time, this scarring can get worse and turn into cirrhosis, which makes it really hard for the liver to do its job. Cirrhosis can even lead to liver failure or liver cancer.

Knowing how liver diseases start can help you take action to stop them early. Regular checkups and healthy habits can make a big difference.

How to Protect and Heal Your Liver

The good news? You can do a lot to keep your liver healthy or help it recover if it's already damaged. Here are some easy ways to take care of your liver:

1. Live a Healthy Lifestyle

Eat well: Choose foods like fruits, veggies, lean meats, and whole grains. Avoid junk food, sugary drinks, and unhealthy fats.

Exercise regularly: Staying active helps you keep a healthy weight and reduces fat in your liver.

Drink less alcohol: Cutting back—or not drinking at all—can prevent liver damage.

2. Protect Yourself from Infections

Get vaccines for hepatitis A and B to stay safe from these common liver infections.

Wash your hands, avoid dirty water, and be careful with sharp objects to avoid getting hepatitis.

3. Get Checkups

Regular blood tests and scans can spot liver problems early, even before you feel sick.

If liver problems run in your family, talk to a doctor about getting tested.

4. Use Medicine When Needed

If you have a liver disease, some medicines can slow it down or even reverse damage.

In serious cases, a liver transplant might be the best option.

This book will teach you more about how your liver works, how to keep it healthy, and what to do if it's not working well. Whether you're learning for yourself or helping a loved one, this guide will make understanding and caring for the liver much easier.

Your journey to better liver health starts here!

PART 1: UNDERSTANDING THE LIVER

CHAPTER 1: THE LIVER'S ROLE IN THE BODY

Key Jobs of a Healthy Liver

Your liver is one of the busiest organs in your body. It does many important jobs to keep you healthy, including:

1. Filtering Toxins: The liver helps clean your blood by getting rid of bad stuff like alcohol, drugs, and toxins.

2. Turning Food into Energy: After you eat, your liver helps break down the food into energy your body can use.

3. **Storing Nutrients and Energy:** Your liver stores important vitamins and minerals, like vitamins A, D, and B12. It also keeps extra sugar (called glycogen) for energy when you need it.

4. **Making Bile:** The liver produces bile, which helps your body digest fat and absorb vitamins.

5. **Making Important Proteins:** The liver makes proteins like albumin, which helps keep the right amount of fluid in your blood, and clotting factors that help your blood clot when you get hurt.

6. **Controlling Blood Sugar:** The liver helps keep your blood sugar levels

stable by storing sugar and releasing it when your body needs it.

7. Regulating Cholesterol: The liver produces cholesterol (a type of fat) needed for building cells and making hormones. It also removes extra cholesterol from your body.

8. Helping Your Immune System: The liver helps your body fight off germs and bacteria by removing them from your blood.

9. Cleaning Up Waste: The liver breaks down harmful chemicals and waste products, like old red blood cells, and helps get rid of them.

How the Liver Affects Your Overall Health

Your liver is important not just for digestion, but for your whole body. A healthy liver helps you feel good, while a sick liver can cause problems. Here's how a healthy liver helps your body:

1. Energy and Vitality: The liver gives you energy by turning food into fuel. If your liver isn't working right, you might feel tired or weak.

2. Mood and Brain Health: The liver helps get rid of toxins, which can affect your brain. If the liver is not working properly, you might feel confused, irritable, or foggy in your mind.

3. **Balanced Hormones:** The liver helps control your hormones. If the liver is sick, it can cause problems with your mood, skin, weight, and even your reproductive health.

4. **Digestion and Absorbing Nutrients:** The liver helps digest food and absorb nutrients. If the liver isn't working well, your body might have trouble getting all the nutrients it needs.

5. **Managing Weight:** The liver helps control metabolism (how your body uses energy). If it's not healthy, you might gain weight or have trouble losing it.

6. Skin Health: When the liver isn't working properly, toxins can build up and show up on your skin as acne or yellowing (jaundice).

7. Immune System: A healthy liver helps your immune system fight off infections. A sick liver can make it harder for your body to stay healthy.

8. Heart Health: The liver helps control blood clotting and keeps your blood vessels in good shape. If it's not working well, it can affect your heart and cause cholesterol problems.

9. Long-Term Health: The liver helps protect you from diseases like diabetes,

high cholesterol, and heart problems. Keeping your liver healthy helps protect your body in the long run.

In short, the liver does more than just process food and filter toxins. It helps you feel energetic, keeps your brain sharp, supports digestion, boosts your immune system, and keeps your body running smoothly. A healthy liver is key to living a happy, active life.

CHAPTER 2: RECOGNIZING LIVER DISEASE

Early Warning Signs and Symptoms

Liver diseases can develop slowly and might not show obvious signs until the liver is really damaged. But noticing early warning signs is important for getting treatment before it gets worse. Here are some common symptoms to watch for:

1. Tiredness: If you feel really tired all the time, even after sleeping well, it

could mean your liver isn't working right.

2. Yellowing of the Skin and Eyes: If your skin or the white parts of your eyes look yellow, it could be a sign your liver isn't cleaning toxins from your body properly.

3. Stomach Pain: If you feel pain or a heavy feeling on the right side of your stomach, it might mean your liver is inflamed or not working well.

4. Swelling in the Belly or Legs: If your stomach or legs swell up, it could be because your liver isn't working properly. This is a serious sign and might mean you have cirrhosis.

5. Dark Urine: If your pee is very dark, it could mean your liver isn't getting rid of waste like it should.

6. Light-Colored Stools: If your poop is pale or clay-colored, it could mean your liver isn't making enough bile, which gives poop its normal color.

7. Loss of Appetite or Feeling Sick: If you feel sick or don't feel like eating, it might be because your liver isn't handling food and toxins well.

8. Losing Weight Without Trying: If you're losing weight without doing anything to make it happen, it could be a sign your liver isn't doing its job of absorbing nutrients from food.

9. Itchy Skin: If your skin itches a lot without a rash, it could mean bile is building up in your skin because your liver isn't processing it properly.

10. Bruising Easily: If you're bruising easily or having trouble stopping bleeding, it could mean your liver isn't making the proteins needed to clot blood.

What Your Symptoms Might Mean

While these symptoms could be caused by liver problems, they don't always mean you have a liver disease. But it's important to talk to a doctor if you notice any of these signs. Here's what some of these symptoms could mean:

1. Tiredness and Weakness: These could be signs of early liver problems, like fatty liver disease or hepatitis. If not treated, these conditions can cause more damage.

2. Yellow Skin and Eyes: If your skin or eyes turn yellow, it could mean you have liver problems like hepatitis or

cirrhosis, where the liver can't process waste properly.

3. Stomach Pain: If you feel pain in your stomach, it could mean the liver is inflamed, or you might have fatty liver disease or liver damage.

4. Swelling in the Belly or Legs: Swelling can happen when the liver gets really damaged and starts scarring, a condition called cirrhosis.

5. Dark Pee and Pale Poop: If your pee is dark and your poop is pale, it might mean your liver isn't making or flowing enough bile, which can happen in liver diseases.

6. Feeling Sick and Losing Appetite: If you feel nauseous or don't want to eat, it could be from liver issues like hepatitis or cirrhosis.

7. Losing Weight Unexplained: If you're losing weight without trying, it could be because your liver isn't processing nutrients correctly, which might be caused by liver disease or even liver cancer.

8. Itchy Skin: If you have itchy skin without a rash, it could be from a buildup of bile acids due to liver problems like cirrhosis.

9. Easy Bruising or Bleeding: If you bruise easily or have trouble stopping bleeding, it could be because your liver isn't making the proteins needed for blood clotting, which is a sign of cirrhosis or liver failure.

If you notice any of these symptoms, it's important to see a doctor. Catching liver problems early can help stop them from getting worse. Your doctor might do tests like blood work, an ultrasound, or even a liver biopsy to figure out what's wrong and how to treat it. By noticing the signs early, you can help protect your liver and stay healthy.

CHAPTER 3: DIAGNOSING LIVER PROBLEMS

Bloodwork and Imaging Tests

When you go to the doctor because you're worried about your liver, they will probably start by giving you some blood tests and images of your liver. These tests help the doctor understand how your liver is doing and if it is healthy. Here's what each test does:

Blood Tests:

Blood tests check how well your liver is working. Here are a few tests your doctor might do:

1. Liver Function Tests (LFTs): These tests check for certain enzymes and proteins in your blood that come from the liver. If the liver is not working well, these levels might be higher than normal. Some of these tests are:

ALT (Alanine Aminotransferase): This enzyme helps break down proteins. If it's high, it could mean your liver is inflamed.

AST (Aspartate Aminotransferase): This enzyme can also show liver damage, but it can be high for other reasons too.

Bilirubin: This substance comes from breaking down red blood cells. High levels can cause your skin and eyes to turn yellow (called jaundice) and can show liver problems.

Albumin: This protein is made by the liver. If it's low, your liver may not be working properly.

Prothrombin Time (PT): This test checks how long it takes for your blood to clot. If the liver isn't making enough clotting proteins, the blood may take longer to clot.

2. Hepatitis Tests: These tests check if you have viruses like hepatitis A, B, or C, which can hurt your liver. If you have a virus, it can cause liver damage and might lead to serious problems if not treated.

3. Liver Enzyme Levels: High levels of enzymes like ALP (alkaline phosphatase) and GGT (gamma-glutamyl transferase) can show problems in the liver or bile ducts.

Imaging Tests:

Imaging tests give pictures of your liver so doctors can see if there are any problems with its size or shape. Here are a few types:

1. **Ultrasound:** This test uses sound waves to make a picture of the liver. It's great for finding liver damage, fatty liver disease, tumors, or cysts. It's usually the first test the doctor will do.

2. **CT Scan (Computed Tomography):** This test takes detailed pictures of the liver and nearby organs. It helps find liver tumors or other issues.

3. **MRI (Magnetic Resonance Imaging):** This test uses magnets and radio waves to create very clear pictures of the liver. It's helpful for finding liver cancer or cirrhosis.

4. Elastography (FibroScan): This is a special type of ultrasound that checks how stiff your liver is. A stiff liver could mean there is scarring, which is a sign of chronic liver disease.

Understanding Biopsies and Other Tests

Sometimes, doctors need even more information to understand your liver's health. They might do a liver biopsy or other tests to get a closer look.

Liver Biopsy:

A liver biopsy is when a doctor takes a small piece of your liver to look at it under a microscope. This helps them see how much damage your liver has. There are a few types of liver biopsies:

1. Percutaneous Biopsy: This is the most common kind. The doctor uses a needle to take a small piece of your liver, usually through your skin on the right side of your belly. It's done with local anesthesia and sometimes an ultrasound to help guide the needle.

2. Transjugular Biopsy: If you can't have a percutaneous biopsy, like if you have problems with blood clotting, the doctor will put the needle in a vein in your neck and guide it to your liver.

3. Laparoscopic Biopsy: This method uses a tiny camera to look inside your belly. The doctor can take a liver sample while also checking for any signs of disease.

The results from a liver biopsy can tell doctors how much liver damage there is, whether there's inflammation, scarring, or cirrhosis, and if liver cancer is a concern.

Other Tests:

1. Endoscopy: This test uses a tube with a camera to look inside your stomach and intestines. It can check for swollen veins in the esophagus, which can happen in people with cirrhosis.

2. CT or MRI-guided Biopsy: Sometimes, the doctor will use a CT scan or MRI to guide the needle during a biopsy to make sure they are taking the sample from the right place.

3. Genetic Tests: If your doctor thinks your liver disease might be genetic (passed down through families), they might test your DNA to look for gene changes that can cause liver problems.

4. Stool Tests: Sometimes, stool (poop) tests are used to check for blood or other signs of liver problems, especially if there are also stomach or digestion issues.

Conclusion

To find out if your liver is healthy, doctors use a mix of blood tests, imaging tests, and sometimes liver biopsies. Catching liver problems early is important because it helps prevent further damage. If you have symptoms of liver disease or are at risk, it's important to see a doctor who can recommend the right tests to help you take care of your liver.

PART 2: COMMON LIVER CONDITIONS

CHAPTER 4: NON-ALCOHOLIC FATTY LIVER DISEASE (NAFLD)

What Is NAFLD?

Non-Alcoholic Fatty Liver Disease (NAFLD) happens when too much fat builds up in your liver, but it's not caused by drinking alcohol. This extra fat can harm your liver over time and lead to more serious problems like liver inflammation, scarring, or even liver cancer.

It's normal for your liver to have a small amount of fat, but too much fat can be harmful. NAFLD usually happens because your liver can't break down the fat properly. The exact cause isn't fully known, but it's often linked to lifestyle choices like poor eating habits, not exercising enough, or being overweight. The good news is, if you catch it early, you can make changes to your lifestyle to help stop the problem or even reverse it.

Risk Factors and Symptoms

NAFLD doesn't usually cause obvious symptoms at first. People often don't know they have it until it's discovered during a check-up, when doctors find things like high liver enzymes in blood tests or fat in the liver on an ultrasound.

Risk Factors for NAFLD:

1. Obesity (Being Overweight): If you have too much body fat, it's more likely that fat will build up in your liver.

2. Type 2 Diabetes: If you have high blood sugar levels, it can lead to more fat in your liver.

3. Metabolic Syndrome: This includes things like high blood pressure, high cholesterol, high blood sugar, and extra

belly fat, which all make NAFLD more likely.

4. Poor Diet: Eating lots of unhealthy foods like sugary drinks, fast food, and snacks can cause fat to build up in your liver.

5. High Cholesterol or High Triglycerides: High levels of fat in your blood can also lead to fat in the liver.

6. Family History: If other people in your family have NAFLD, you might be more likely to get it too.

7. Age: NAFLD is more common in middle-aged people, but younger people can have it, especially if they're overweight or have other risk factors.

8. Gender: Men are more likely to get NAFLD, but women might develop it after menopause.

Symptoms of NAFLD:

At first, you might not feel anything. Some people might feel tired or have mild pain in the upper right part of their belly. It can also be found during blood tests or ultrasounds. If it gets worse, though, it might cause:

Jaundice (yellowing of the skin or eyes)

Swollen belly or legs

Dark urine

Easy bruising or bleeding

Confusion or forgetfulness (if the liver is very damaged)

Lifestyle Strategies for Reversal

The good news is that NAFLD can often be helped or even reversed by making some healthy changes in your life. Here are some tips to improve your liver health:

1. Lose Weight:

Losing weight is one of the best ways to reduce liver fat. Even losing just 5-10% of your body weight can make a big difference.

Focus on healthy eating and exercise to lose weight slowly (about 1-2 pounds per week) so it doesn't put too much stress on your liver.

2. Eat a Healthy Diet:

Eat more whole foods like fruits, vegetables, whole grains, and lean proteins.

Choose healthy fats, like those from olive oil, avocados, nuts, and fish, instead of unhealthy fats like those in fried foods and junk food.

Cut down on sugar and processed foods (like soda, candy, and fast food) because they can cause fat to build up in your liver.

Try eating smaller meals throughout the day to keep your blood sugar steady.

3. Exercise Regularly:

Exercising helps burn fat and lowers the fat in your liver. Aim for at least 30 minutes of exercise most days, like walking, biking, or swimming.

Doing both aerobic exercises (like running) and strength training (like lifting weights) is great for your liver.

4. Manage Diabetes and High Cholesterol:

If you have diabetes or high cholesterol, it's important to keep them under control, as they can make NAFLD worse.

Talk to your doctor about how to manage these conditions, and you may need medications to help.

5. Limit Alcohol and Avoid Toxins:

Even though NAFLD isn't caused by alcohol, drinking alcohol can make liver problems worse. It's best to limit alcohol or avoid it.

Be careful with over-the-counter medicines, supplements, or herbs, as some of them can harm your liver. Always ask your doctor before trying new medicines.

6. Get Regular Check-ups:

If you have risk factors for NAFLD, regular check-ups with your doctor are important. They might do blood tests or imaging to see how your liver is doing and make sure the problem doesn't get worse.

Conclusion:

Non-Alcoholic Fatty Liver Disease (NAFLD) is a common liver problem that can often be reversed by making healthy lifestyle changes. By eating better, exercising, losing weight, and managing other health problems like diabetes, you can help your liver get healthier and prevent serious damage. If you think you might be at risk for NAFLD, talk to your doctor about getting checked. Early action and good habits can make a big difference in keeping your liver and overall health in good shape.

CHAPTER 5: ALCOHOL-RELATED LIVER DISEASE (ARLD)

How Alcohol Affects Your Liver

Drinking too much alcohol over a long time can hurt your liver. The liver helps break down alcohol, but it can only handle so much at once. If you drink too much, the liver can get overwhelmed, which can cause damage.

The liver can fix itself a little, but if someone keeps drinking a lot, it can get inflamed, scarred, and might even stop working properly. Alcohol-related liver disease (ARLD) happens when alcohol causes liver damage. It can happen to anyone who drinks a lot, but some people are at a higher risk because of things like their genes, diet, or other health problems.

The Stages of ARLD: Fatty Liver, Hepatitis, and Cirrhosis

ARLD has three stages, and each one gets more serious than the last. These stages are fatty liver, alcoholic hepatitis, and cirrhosis.

1. Fatty Liver:

This is the first stage and happens when too much fat builds up in the liver from drinking too much alcohol.

You usually don't feel anything in this stage, but it can turn into something worse if you keep drinking. The good news is that fatty liver can be fixed by drinking less alcohol and eating better.

2. Alcoholic Hepatitis:

This is when your liver becomes inflamed because of alcohol.

It can make you feel sick with symptoms like yellow skin or eyes (called jaundice), fever, stomach pain, and not feeling hungry.

Alcoholic hepatitis can be mild or really serious. If you stop drinking, your liver can heal, but if you keep drinking, it can cause permanent damage.

3. Cirrhosis:

This is the worst stage of ARLD, where your liver gets so damaged that it forms scars.

Cirrhosis can make the liver stop working properly, which can cause problems like bleeding or liver failure.

Once you have cirrhosis, the damage can't be fixed, but with the right care, you can manage it and stop it from getting worse.

How to Treat and Recover from ARLD

If ARLD is found early, it's possible to slow down or even fix some of the damage with the right treatment and by making some changes in your life. The most important thing to do is stop drinking alcohol completely. If you keep drinking, the damage will only get worse.

Here are some steps to help treat ARLD:

1. Stop Drinking Alcohol:

The most important thing is to stop drinking alcohol. This lets your liver start healing and stops it from getting worse.

If you've been drinking heavily, a doctor might suggest a program to help you safely stop and deal with withdrawal symptoms.

2. Eat Healthy:

Eating a balanced diet helps your liver heal. People with liver disease often don't get enough nutrients, so it's important to eat foods like fruits, vegetables, lean meats, and whole grains.

A doctor might also suggest vitamins if you're missing any important nutrients.

3. Medications:

If you have alcoholic hepatitis, doctors can give you medicine to reduce inflammation or help with symptoms.

If cirrhosis happens, other medicines may be needed to treat complications like swelling, infections, or bleeding. In really bad cases, a liver transplant may be needed.

4. Regular Checkups:

If you have ARLD, you need to see a doctor regularly. Blood tests, ultrasounds, or other tests can check how your liver is doing and catch problems early.

Your doctor will also help you manage other health issues like high blood pressure or diabetes.

5. Support and Counseling:

Recovering from ARLD can be tough, especially if you have a problem with alcohol. Support groups or therapy can help you stay sober and deal with any emotional struggles.

Counseling can also help you understand why you drink and teach you ways to handle cravings or difficult situations.

6. Liver Transplant (in Severe Cases):

If your liver is so damaged that it stops working and other treatments aren't working, you might need a liver transplant. This is a surgery where a healthy liver from a donor replaces your damaged one.

Not everyone can get a transplant, so doctors will check if it's the right choice for you.

Conclusion

Alcohol-related liver disease (ARLD) is serious and can cause long-term liver damage. It starts with fatty liver, then can turn into alcoholic hepatitis, and finally cirrhosis, the most serious stage. The first step in recovery is to stop drinking alcohol completely. With the right care, healthy habits, and support, you can manage ARLD, protect your liver, and even prevent it from getting worse. If you think you might have ARLD, it's really important to see a doctor and start treatment early to give your liver the best chance to heal.

CHAPTER 6: HEPATITIS

What is Hepatitis?

Hepatitis is when your liver gets inflamed, often because of a virus. The liver is an important organ that helps your body clean out toxins and digest food. There are different types of hepatitis, each caused by different viruses. The main types are Hepatitis A, B, C, D, and E.

1. Hepatitis A:
Hepatitis A is a virus that spreads through contaminated food or water. It's more common in places with poor

hygiene. This type usually doesn't cause long-term liver problems and can go away on its own. It can cause fever, tiredness, stomach pain, and yellow skin or eyes (called jaundice).

2. Hepatitis B:
Hepatitis B is spread through contact with infected blood or body fluids, like during unprotected sex or from sharing needles. Some people get better on their own, but others can get a long-term (chronic) infection that might harm the liver over time, leading to serious problems like cirrhosis or liver cancer.

3. Hepatitis C:
Hepatitis C is mostly spread through blood. It's commonly spread by sharing needles or receiving tainted blood.

Most people with Hepatitis C get a long-term infection, which can cause liver damage and even need a liver transplant.

4. Hepatitis D:
Hepatitis D can only happen if someone already has Hepatitis B. It makes the Hepatitis B infection worse, leading to even more liver damage. It spreads through blood and body fluids, and can lead to more serious liver problems.

5. Hepatitis E:
Hepatitis E is spread through contaminated water, especially in places with poor sanitation. Most people recover without any long-term

problems, but it can be very serious for pregnant women, possibly causing liver failure.

Causes, Symptoms, and Treatments

1. Causes:

Hepatitis A is caused by eating or drinking contaminated food or water.

Hepatitis B and D spread through contact with infected blood or body fluids.

Hepatitis C spreads through blood-to-blood contact.

Hepatitis E is caused by drinking contaminated water.

2. Symptoms: Hepatitis might not show any symptoms at first, but later it can cause:

Feeling very tired (fatigue)

Yellow skin or eyes (jaundice)

Pain in the belly, especially on the right side

Feeling sick to your stomach, throwing up, or not feeling hungry

Dark urine and light-colored stools

Fever and pain in your joints

3. Treatment:

Hepatitis A: No special medicine is needed for Hepatitis A. Most people get better on their own by resting and drinking plenty of fluids. There's a vaccine to prevent it.

Hepatitis B: Some people recover by themselves, but others need medicine to manage the infection. There's also a vaccine to prevent it.

Hepatitis C: There are medicines that can cure Hepatitis C. These medications usually last a few months, and many people get better.

Hepatitis D: Treatment focuses on managing Hepatitis B, since you need it to get Hepatitis D. Medicines might help control it.

Hepatitis E: Most people get better without treatment, but pregnant women or people with weak immune systems may need special medicine.

How to Prevent Hepatitis

1. Vaccination:

You can get vaccines for Hepatitis A and B, which can protect you from these types. There's no vaccine for Hepatitis C, D, or E, but there are ways to reduce the risk of getting them.

2. Safe Practices:

Hepatitis A: Wash your hands often, especially before eating or cooking. Drink clean, safe water, especially when traveling to places where water sanitation is poor.

Hepatitis B, C, and D: Don't share things like needles, razors, or toothbrushes. Make sure any tattoos or piercings are done with clean equipment. Practice safe sex by using condoms.

Hepatitis E: Drink clean water and avoid eating undercooked meat, especially pork or deer, if you're in an area where Hepatitis E is common.

3. Testing and Early Detection:

If you're at risk, like if you've shared needles or had unprotected sex, get tested for hepatitis. Early testing helps find it before it causes serious problems.

4. Good Hygiene:

For Hepatitis A and E, since they spread through dirty water and food, always wash your hands, especially after using the bathroom or before eating. Drink safe water and eat clean food.

Conclusion

Hepatitis is a disease that can seriously affect your liver, but it's important to know how it spreads, how to protect yourself, and what to do if you get it. Vaccines can help prevent Hepatitis A and B, and good hygiene can protect against A and E. Hepatitis B, C, and D spread through blood and body fluids, so safe practices are key to prevention. If you're at risk, make sure to get tested and take care of your liver health.

CHAPTER 7: CIRRHOSIS

What is Cirrhosis?

Cirrhosis happens when the liver, a vital organ in your body, gets damaged over time and is replaced by scar tissue. The liver helps your body by cleaning out bad stuff, breaking down food, and making bile to help digest fats. When the liver is damaged, it can't do these jobs properly, which can cause health problems.

Cirrhosis usually happens after many years of damage to the liver. At first, you might not feel anything wrong, but as the liver gets more damaged, serious problems can happen.

What Causes Cirrhosis and What Can It Do?

Cirrhosis can be caused by different things. Some common causes include:

1. Drinking Too Much Alcohol: Drinking a lot of alcohol over many years can hurt the liver and cause scarring.

2. Chronic Hepatitis (Liver Infection): Hepatitis B and C are infections that hurt the liver and can cause cirrhosis if not treated.

3. Non-Alcoholic Fatty Liver Disease (NAFLD): This happens when too much fat builds up in the liver, often because of being overweight or having diabetes. It can cause cirrhosis if not taken care of.

4. Autoimmune Hepatitis: This happens when the body's immune system attacks the liver by mistake, causing damage.

5. Genetic Problems: Some people inherit diseases that affect the liver, like too much iron or copper in the liver.

6. Medications and Toxins: Taking too many medicines or being exposed to

harmful chemicals can hurt the liver over time.

As cirrhosis gets worse, it can lead to serious health problems, like:

Liver Cancer: Scar tissue in the liver can make it easier to get liver cancer.

Portal Hypertension: Too much pressure in the liver's blood vessels can cause bleeding in the stomach or throat.

Ascites: Fluid can build up in the belly, causing it to swell and hurt.

Encephalopathy: If the liver can't clean out toxins, it can affect the brain, causing confusion or changes in behavior.

Liver Failure: When the liver stops working, it can cause life-threatening problems.

How to Manage Cirrhosis

Even though cirrhosis can't be fully cured, you can manage it and stop it from getting worse. The goal is to protect the liver, reduce symptoms, and prevent other problems.

1. Fix the Cause:

If alcohol caused the cirrhosis, stop drinking alcohol.

If hepatitis caused it, medicines can help fight the infection.

If fatty liver disease is the cause, eating healthier and losing weight can help.

If it's autoimmune hepatitis, medicines to calm the immune system can reduce damage.

2. Medications: Some medicines can help protect the liver and treat problems caused by cirrhosis, like fluid buildup or bleeding.

3. Healthy Lifestyle:

Eat Well: A healthy diet is very important. Avoid too much salt, sugar, and fat to give your liver less stress. If there's fluid in the belly, eating less salt helps.

Exercise: Being active helps your body and can improve liver health.

Avoid Harmful Substances: Stay away from alcohol, some medications, and harmful chemicals.

4. Regular Check-ups: Getting regular blood tests helps doctors check how well the liver is working. People with cirrhosis should also get checked for liver cancer, especially if their cirrhosis is caused by hepatitis or alcohol.

5. Liver Transplant: In some cases, when the liver is too damaged, getting a liver transplant (a new liver from someone else) might be needed.

Conclusion

Cirrhosis is a serious liver disease caused by long-term damage, but with proper care, it can often be controlled. Stopping the cause of the damage, taking medicines, and making healthy lifestyle changes can help slow down the disease. If you or someone you know has cirrhosis, it's important to work with a doctor to manage it and stay as healthy as possible.

CHAPTER 8: LIVER CANCER

Liver cancer happens when abnormal cells grow out of control in the liver, which is an important organ in your body. The liver helps with things like digesting food and cleaning toxins out of the body. When liver cancer happens, it can make these functions harder to do. In this chapter, we'll talk about the different types of liver cancer, how to spot the signs, and the treatments that can help.

Types of Liver Cancer and What Makes Them Different

There are a few types of liver cancer, and each one behaves a little differently:

1. Hepatocellular Carcinoma (HCC): This is the most common type of liver cancer. It starts in the main cells of the liver and is often caused by liver problems like cirrhosis, hepatitis, or fatty liver disease.

2. Cholangiocarcinoma (Bile Duct Cancer): This type starts in the bile ducts, which carry bile from the liver to

the gallbladder and small intestine. It's less common and harder to catch early.

3. Liver Angiosarcoma: This is a rare, fast-growing cancer that starts in the blood vessels of the liver. It's usually diagnosed later because it doesn't always show symptoms right away.

4. Hepatoblastoma: This is a rare liver cancer that mostly affects young children. It grows quickly but can be treated, and many kids with this cancer can survive.

Each type of liver cancer needs different treatments, so it's important to know which type you have.

Early Signs and How to Detect Liver Cancer

Liver cancer can be hard to find early because its symptoms can be similar to other problems. But noticing signs early can make treatment more successful. Here are some signs to watch out for:

1. Unexplained Weight Loss: Losing weight without trying, especially with a loss of appetite, can be a sign of liver cancer.

2. Tiredness or Weakness: If you feel really tired or weak all the time, even after sleeping well, it could be a sign that your liver isn't working well.

3. Abdominal Pain or Swelling: Pain in the upper right side of your belly or swelling could be caused by a tumor in the liver.

4. Yellow Skin or Eyes (Jaundice): If your skin or the whites of your eyes turn yellow, it might be a sign your liver isn't processing waste properly.

5. Nausea or Vomiting: Feeling sick or throwing up with no clear reason could be related to liver cancer.

6. Itchy Skin: If your skin feels itchy without any obvious reason, it could mean there's a problem with your liver.

How Doctors Find Liver Cancer

There are a few ways doctors can find liver cancer:

1. Imaging Tests:

Ultrasound: This test uses sound waves to create pictures of your liver and can find tumors.

CT Scan: This test creates detailed images of your liver and helps doctors see tumors clearly.

MRI: An MRI gives a more detailed picture of the liver and helps doctors plan treatment.

2. Blood Tests:

==Alpha-Fetoprotein (AFP) Test==: High levels of AFP in the blood can suggest liver cancer, especially if you already have liver disease.

Liver Function Tests: These tests check how well your liver is working by measuring certain substances in your blood.

3. Biopsy: A doctor might remove a small piece of the liver to test it for cancer cells. This helps confirm the diagnosis.

Treatment Options for Liver Cancer

The treatment for liver cancer depends on many things, like how bad the cancer is and how healthy the liver is. Here are some treatments that might be used:

1. Surgery:

Liver Resection: If the tumor is only in one part of the liver and the liver is still healthy, doctors might remove the tumor.

Liver Transplant: If the liver is too damaged or the tumor is too big to remove, a liver transplant might be needed. This means getting a healthy liver from a donor.

2. Ablation Therapy: These treatments use heat or chemicals to destroy the cancer cells:

Radiofrequency Ablation (RFA): This uses heat to burn the cancer cells.

Percutaneous Ethanol Injection (PEI): This injects alcohol into the tumor to kill the cancer cells.

3. Chemotherapy: This uses medicine to kill cancer cells, but liver cancer can be hard to treat with chemotherapy alone.

4. Targeted Therapy: This focuses on blocking things that help cancer grow. Some drugs can target specific molecules to stop the cancer from spreading.

5. Immunotherapy: This type of treatment helps your body's immune system fight the cancer.

6. Radiation Therapy: Radiation uses strong energy to kill cancer cells. It's used if surgery isn't an option or if cancer has spread.

Conclusion

Liver cancer is serious, but if it's found early, it can be treated. If you or someone you know has liver problems, it's important to see a doctor regularly and watch for any signs of cancer. With the right treatment, many people with liver cancer can live longer and feel better. Always talk to your doctor to find out the best treatment for your specific situation.

PART 3: LIVER-FRIENDLY DIET AND NUTRITION

CHAPTER 9: THE ROLE OF DIET IN LIVER HEALTH

Your liver is a very important organ in your body. It helps clean your blood, turn food into energy, and store nutrients. Even though your liver is strong and can heal itself, it needs help from a good diet to stay healthy. What you eat can either help or harm your liver, so it's important to know how nutrition affects it. In this chapter, we'll talk about how your diet influences liver health and which foods can help your liver stay strong.

How Nutrition Affects the Liver

The foods you eat affect how well your liver works. The liver processes everything you eat and drink, so if you eat healthy foods, your liver can do its job better. But if you eat too many junk foods, it can make your liver sick and lead to problems like fatty liver disease or liver inflammation.

Here's how what you eat can affect your liver:

1. Fatty Liver Disease: Eating too many unhealthy fats, like those in fried foods or junk food, can cause fat to build up in the liver, which can make it sick over time.

2. Inflammation: A diet full of processed foods, sugar, and alcohol can make your liver swollen and inflamed, which can lead to liver problems.

3. Detoxification: Eating healthy foods with lots of vitamins, minerals, and antioxidants helps your liver clean out toxins and keep your body healthy.

4. Liver Repair: Some foods help your liver heal when it's damaged, so it's important to eat the right nutrients to help it recover.

A healthy diet can keep your liver working well and even help it heal if it's been damaged.

Foods to Support Liver Function

If you want to take care of your liver, you need to eat foods that reduce swelling, help clean out toxins, and give your liver the nutrients it needs. Here are some foods that help your liver stay healthy:

1. Leafy Greens: Vegetables like spinach, kale, and dandelion greens help your liver clean toxins from your blood.

2. Cruciferous Vegetables: Broccoli, cauliflower, Brussels sprouts, and cabbage help your liver make the enzymes it needs to get rid of toxins.

3. Garlic: Garlic helps your liver work better by activating the enzymes that clean out toxins. It also helps reduce inflammation.

4. Beets: Beets have special nutrients that help your liver process toxins and improve blood flow.

5. Berries: Blueberries, strawberries, and raspberries have antioxidants that protect your liver from damage and help it heal.

6. Nuts and Seeds: Almonds, walnuts, and flaxseeds are full of healthy fats and vitamin E, which help reduce liver inflammation and protect it from damage.

7. Turmeric: This yellow spice has curcumin, which helps protect the liver, reduce inflammation, and help it heal.

8. Green Tea: Green tea has antioxidants that help your liver work better and protect it from damage.

9. Avocados: Avocados are full of healthy fats that help your liver work well and protect it from stress.

10. Lemon and Citrus Fruits: Lemons, grapefruits, and oranges are full of vitamin C, which helps your liver clean out toxins. The acid in lemons also helps your liver make bile, which is important for digestion.

11. Olive Oil: Olive oil has healthy fats that can reduce liver fat and inflammation. It also helps your liver work better.

Foods to Limit for Liver Health

While some foods help your liver, others can harm it. To keep your liver healthy, try to eat less of these foods:

Alcohol: Drinking too much alcohol can hurt your liver and cause liver disease.

Processed Foods: Foods like chips, candy, and fast food have too much sugar and unhealthy fats that can harm your liver.

Fried Foods: Foods that are fried in unhealthy oils can put stress on your liver.

Red Meat: Eating too much red meat, like burgers or steak, can make your liver work too hard.

Conclusion

To keep your liver healthy, it's important to eat the right foods. Leafy greens, broccoli, garlic, berries, and healthy fats like those in avocados and olive oil are great for liver health. On the other hand, eating too many unhealthy foods, like junk food and alcohol, can harm your liver. By choosing healthier foods, you can help your liver do its job and keep your body strong.

CHAPTER 10: FOODS TO AVOID FOR A HEALTHY LIVER

Your liver is super important for keeping your body healthy, and one of the best ways to help it stay strong is by avoiding foods that can hurt it. Some foods are good for your liver, but others can cause damage, make it harder to work, and even lead to serious diseases. In this chapter, we'll talk about which foods and habits to avoid and give some tips for eating risky foods in a safer way.

Foods and Habits That Harm the Liver

Some foods and habits are really tough on your liver and can hurt it if you have them too often. Here are some things that can cause liver problems:

1. Alcohol Alcohol can hurt your liver. When your liver breaks down alcohol, it makes toxic stuff that can inflame and damage the liver. Drinking a lot over time can lead to serious liver problems.

Tip: If you drink alcohol, keep it to special occasions and follow the rules: no more than one drink per day for women and two for men.

2. Processed Foods Processed foods, like fast food, chips, cookies, and frozen meals, often have too much sugar, fat, and chemicals. These can make your liver work too hard and cause fat to build up, which isn't good for it.

Tip: Eat more fresh foods like vegetables, fruits, lean meats, and whole grains. Try to keep processed foods for special treats, not every day.

3. Trans Fats Trans fats are unhealthy fats found in lots of packaged foods. They can cause liver inflammation and fat buildup.

Tip: Avoid foods with "hydrogenated oils" or "partially hydrogenated oils" on the label. Choose healthier oils like olive oil or avocado oil.

4. Refined Sugars and High-Fructose Corn Syrup Sugars in sodas, candy, and sugary snacks can quickly turn into fat in the liver. Too much sugar can lead to fatty liver disease and other problems.

Tip: Try to cut back on sugary drinks and candy. Eat natural sweets like fruits, and check food labels for hidden sugars.

5. Fried Foods Fried foods, like french fries and fried chicken, have unhealthy fats that can damage your liver. They cause liver inflammation and fat buildup.

Tip: Avoid fried foods as much as possible. Try cooking with healthy oils like olive oil, or bake, grill, or steam your food instead.

6. Red Meat and Fatty Meats Red meats like beef, sausages, and burgers can put a lot of stress on your liver. They have unhealthy fats that can build up in the liver and cause problems.

Tip: Limit red meat to only a few times a week. Choose lean meats like chicken or fish instead. Plant-based foods like beans and tofu are also great options.

7. Salt and High-Sodium Foods Too much salt, found in processed foods like chips and canned soups, can make

it harder for your liver to do its job. It can also lead to high blood pressure.

Tip: Use less salt and choose fresh, whole foods. You can add flavor with herbs and spices instead of salt.

8. Artificial Additives and Food Colorings Many processed foods have artificial chemicals and colorings that can build up in your liver over time, causing harm.

Tip: Eat more fresh foods and avoid processed ones with artificial chemicals. Look for foods with short ingredient lists and no artificial colors.

Moderation Tips for Risky Foods

Some foods are okay to eat sometimes but not every day. Here's how you can enjoy them without hurting your liver:

1. Alcohol: If you drink, keep it to one drink per day for women and two for men. Take breaks from alcohol to give your liver rest.

2. Red Meat: You don't have to cut out red meat, but try to have it only once or twice a week. Pick lean cuts like sirloin or try turkey.

3. Processed Foods: Processed foods can be unhealthy, so only eat them now and then. Cooking at home lets you control what goes into your food.

4. Fried Foods: Fried foods are not great for your liver. Have them only on special occasions and cook your meals in healthier ways like grilling or baking.

5. Sugar: It's hard to give up sugar, but try to limit sugary drinks and snacks. Aim for no more than 25 grams of sugar per day.

6. Salt: Too much salt can hurt your liver, so use it sparingly. Try using

herbs, spices, and other flavorings instead of salt.

Conclusion

The foods you eat can affect your liver health. By avoiding alcohol, processed foods, unhealthy fats, sugar, and too much salt, you can help keep your liver healthy. Some of these foods can be okay if eaten in moderation, but try to keep them as occasional treats. Making good food choices will help protect your liver from damage and keep it working well for you.

CHAPTER 11: MEAL PLANS AND RECIPES

Eating healthy foods is really important for keeping your liver strong and helping it heal if it's not feeling well. In this chapter, we'll share some meal ideas and easy recipes that can help your liver stay healthy and recover.

Liver-Friendly Meal Ideas

Here are some meal ideas that are good for your liver:

1. Breakfast Ideas:

Oatmeal with Berries and Chia Seeds: Oats are great for digestion, berries help fight inflammation, and chia seeds give you healthy fats and fiber.

Green Smoothie: Blend spinach, kale, cucumber, apple, and flaxseeds. These are full of vitamins that help your liver.

2. Lunch Ideas:

Grilled Chicken Salad with Avocado: A simple salad with grilled chicken, greens, and avocado. The chicken gives you protein, and avocado is full of healthy fats.

Quinoa and Roasted Vegetables: Quinoa is a good plant-based protein, and roasted vegetables like sweet potatoes and carrots help protect your liver.

3. Dinner Ideas:

Salmon with Steamed Veggies: Salmon is full of omega-3 fats that help reduce liver problems. Pair it with steamed vegetables like broccoli and carrots.

Lentil and Spinach Soup: Lentils are packed with protein and fiber, while spinach helps the liver detox.

4. Snack Ideas:

Apple Slices with Almond Butter: Apples are full of fiber and antioxidants, and almond butter gives you healthy fats and protein.

Carrot and Celery Sticks with Hummus: Carrots and celery are low in calories and help digestion. Hummus is a tasty dip that has protein.

Recipes to Help Your Liver Recover

Here are some tasty and simple recipes to help your liver heal:

1. Turmeric and Ginger Smoothie

Ingredients: Coconut milk, banana, turmeric powder, fresh ginger, chia seeds, black pepper, ice cubes.

How to Make It: Blend all the ingredients together. Enjoy this smoothie for breakfast or a snack.

Why It's Good for Your Liver: Turmeric and ginger help reduce inflammation and support your liver.

2. Lemon Garlic Salmon

Ingredients: Salmon fillets, garlic, lemon, olive oil, salt, pepper, parsley.

How to Make It: Preheat the oven, mix garlic, lemon, olive oil, salt, and pepper, and brush over the salmon. Bake for 15-20 minutes and serve with vegetables or quinoa.

Why It's Good for Your Liver: Salmon is full of omega-3 fatty acids that help the liver, and garlic helps protect the liver.

3. Detoxifying Lentil and Vegetable Soup

Ingredients: Lentils, olive oil, onion, garlic, carrots, celery, zucchini, tomatoes, vegetable broth, turmeric, cumin, salt, pepper, parsley.

How to Make It: Heat olive oil, sauté onions and garlic, add vegetables, lentils, broth, and spices. Simmer for 25-30 minutes and serve with parsley.

Why It's Good for Your Liver: Lentils provide fiber and protein, and turmeric and cumin help reduce liver inflammation.

4. Avocado and Chickpea Salad

Ingredients: Avocado, chickpeas, cucumber, red onion, olive oil, lemon juice, salt, pepper, cilantro.

How to Make It: Mix avocado, chickpeas, cucumber, and onion in a bowl. Add olive oil and lemon juice, then toss and garnish with cilantro.

Why It's Good for Your Liver: Avocados have healthy fats, and chickpeas provide fiber and protein, both helping your liver.

Conclusion

Eating liver-friendly meals is a great way to support your liver and help it recover. Focus on eating whole, natural foods like fruits, vegetables, lean meats, and healthy fats. Delicious recipes like turmeric smoothies, lemon garlic salmon, lentil soups, and avocado salads are easy ways to give your liver the nutrients it needs to stay strong and heal. A healthy diet is an important part of taking care of your liver and preventing liver problems.

CONCLUSION

Taking care of your liver is essential for maintaining overall health, as the liver plays a critical role in detoxifying the body, processing nutrients, and supporting various bodily functions. Liver diseases, such as fatty liver, hepatitis, and cirrhosis, can greatly affect your quality of life, but with the right knowledge, lifestyle changes, and medical care, it's possible to manage, prevent, and even reverse liver damage.

Throughout this book, we've discussed the importance of liver health, the causes and symptoms of liver disease, and how to support your liver through diet, exercise, and medical care. By following the practical tips outlined here, such as eating liver-friendly foods, avoiding alcohol, managing weight, and getting regular check-ups, you can help your liver function optimally and reduce the risk of disease. Remember, taking small but consistent steps toward a healthier lifestyle can make a big difference in your liver health.

Practical Steps to Protect Your Liver

Taking care of your liver doesn't have to be complicated. Here are some simple, practical steps you can take every day to protect your liver:

1. Maintain a Healthy Diet:

Focus on whole, nutrient-dense foods like vegetables, fruits, whole grains, and lean proteins.

Include liver-supporting foods like leafy greens, berries, fatty fish, nuts, and seeds.

Avoid processed foods high in sugar, salt, and unhealthy fats.

2. Exercise Regularly:

Aim for at least 30 minutes of moderate physical activity most days of the week. Regular exercise helps maintain a healthy weight, improves metabolism, and supports liver health.

3. Avoid Excessive Alcohol:

Drinking too much alcohol can overwhelm the liver and cause damage. If you drink, do so in moderation, and if possible, limit alcohol consumption or avoid it altogether.

4. Manage Weight:

Excess weight, especially belly fat, can lead to fatty liver disease. Eating a balanced diet and staying active can help maintain a healthy weight.

5. Stay Hydrated:

Drink plenty of water throughout the day to help your liver flush out toxins and maintain overall health.

6. Avoid Toxins:

Limit exposure to chemicals, pollutants, and toxins that can harm the liver. This includes avoiding unnecessary medications, quitting smoking, and reducing exposure to harmful environmental substances.

7. Get Regular Check-Ups:

Regular visits to your doctor can help detect liver problems early. Your healthcare provider can perform tests like blood work and ultrasounds to check liver function and screen for any potential issues.

8. Take Care of Your Mental Health:

Stress can negatively affect liver health, so make sure to take time for relaxation, mindfulness, and activities that make you happy.

Innovations in Liver Disease Management

Medical advancements in liver disease treatment have made significant progress, offering new hope for people living with liver conditions. Here are some of the latest innovations in liver disease management:

1. Non-Invasive Tests for Liver Health:

Traditional liver biopsies are being replaced by non-invasive tests, such as elastography and blood biomarkers, which can measure liver stiffness and detect liver damage more safely and accurately. These tests help doctors monitor liver disease progression without the need for invasive procedures.

2. Gene Therapy:

Gene therapy is an emerging treatment that aims to treat liver diseases at the genetic level. This involves replacing or repairing defective genes that cause liver problems, potentially offering a cure for certain genetic liver disorders.

3. Stem Cell Therapy:

Stem cell therapy has shown promise in regenerating damaged liver tissue. Researchers are investigating how stem cells can help repair liver cells, offering hope for people with cirrhosis and other forms of liver damage.

4. Advanced Medications:

New drugs are being developed to treat chronic liver diseases like hepatitis B and C, as well as fatty liver disease. These medications help reduce inflammation, fight viral infections, and support liver function, often with fewer side effects than older treatments.

5. Liver Transplantation Advances:

Liver transplantation has seen major improvements, including better matching techniques, improved immunosuppressive drugs to prevent rejection, and more successful transplant outcomes. There is also progress in living-donor liver transplants, where a portion of a healthy person's liver is transplanted into a patient.

6. Artificial Liver Devices:

In cases of acute liver failure, artificial liver devices are being developed to temporarily support liver function while the liver heals or while a transplant is being arranged. These devices help bridge the gap between liver failure and recovery or transplant.

7. Personalized Medicine:

As we learn more about the genetic and molecular causes of liver diseases, treatments are becoming more personalized. This means doctors can offer therapies tailored to a person's specific condition, increasing the chances of success and reducing side effects.

8. Fatty Liver Disease Treatments:

New drugs and therapies for non-alcoholic fatty liver disease (NAFLD) and non-alcoholic steatohepatitis

(NASH) are being researched. These treatments focus on reducing liver fat, improving liver function, and preventing complications like cirrhosis.

Final Thoughts

Caring for your liver is an ongoing process, and the journey to better liver health starts with understanding the role of the liver in your body and the steps you can take to protect it. By maintaining a healthy diet, staying active, avoiding toxins, and seeking medical care when needed, you can safeguard your liver and support its natural healing process.

In the future, as medical science continues to advance, even more effective treatments and interventions for liver diseases will emerge. But for now, by making small, consistent changes in your lifestyle and following the latest innovations in treatment, you can take control of your liver health and live a long, healthy life.

Your liver is a vital organ that deserves care and attention. With the right steps, you can give your liver the support it needs to thrive.

Made in the USA
Middletown, DE
15 May 2025

75604527R00076